365 Daze

Lesa Kelley Osborn

authorHOUSE®

AuthorHouse™
1663 Liberty Drive
Bloomington, IN 47403
www.authorhouse.com
Phone: 1-800-839-8640

First published by AuthorHouse 05/11/2011
Rev. 10/8/12

ISBN: 978-1-4567-4573-8 (e)
ISBN: 978-1-4567-4572-1 (sc)

Library of Congress Control Number: 2011903912
Printed in the United States of America

ACKNOWLEDGEMENTS

To the best parents and brother anyone could ask for:
Thank you for your love and support.

To Alex and Tristen:
You are the joy in my life.

To my close friends who talked me
through the toughest times:
Thank you from the bottom of my heart.

To Sallie Boyles whose talents and
encouragement motivated me to
completion of this project.

To my friends at *Network Communications,
Inc.* who took time from their busy schedule
to stop by my office with kind words.

And to God, who never left me, even when I
was too distraught to acknowledge him.

DEDICATION

This book is dedicated to *the overwhelmed*.

CONTENTS

CHAPTER ONE
The Call 1

CHAPTER TWO
The Boyfriend 11

CHAPTER THREE
Clueless 21

CHAPTER FOUR
Overwhelmed 29

CHAPTER FIVE
Beautiful Strangers 39

CHAPTER SIX
Midst Of Chaos 47

CHAPTER SEVEN
Freak Show 59

CHAPTER EIGHT
The Note 67

CHAPTER NINE
Déjà vu 77

CHAPTER TEN
Blue Eyes 85

CHAPTER ONE

The Call

"Don't worry about the future, but know that worrying is as effective as trying to solve an algebra equation by chewing bubble gum. The real troubles in your life are apt to be things that never crossed your worried mind, the kind that blindside you at 4 p.m. on some idle Tuesday." – Mary Schmich

My Tuesday morning drive to the office in the Atlanta burbs was like any other. Driving down Satellite Boulevard to company headquarters, I made my commute in its usual twenty-five minutes. Without incident, I wheeled my silver SUV into the same crowded parking lot and then entered the familiar two-story, stucco office building as I had day after day. I could have closed my eyes and walked through the lobby and known when to stop at the elevator door by counting the number of heel-toe taps my shoes made on the marble.

Once on the second floor, I made my predictable detour to the dimly lit break room. Easing into a work mode, I poured my ritual mug before taking the last leg of my early morning trek to my office down the hall. Settling at my desk, I was about to take a sip when, as if on cue, my cell phone rang.

"Hello?" I answered without a second thought.

"Hi, this is Dr. Auda's office. Is this Lesa?" the woman asked.

"Yes." I replied.

"Dr. Auda needs to speak with you. Can you hold?"

"Yes, I can hold." I said

I had been in Dr. Auda's office five days earlier for a mammogram. After I showed my gynecologist what felt to be a golf ball-sized lump in my left breast, he referred me to Dr. Auda, a respected breast health specialist. To me, Dr. Auda's head of thick white hair, small stature and easygoing manner made him seem more like a gentle grandfather than a top surgeon.

Maybe it was a combination of his temperament and my here-we-go-again assumptions, but the sequence of events during that visit barely fazed me. First, Dr. Auda ordered a second mammogram, which took place immediately after he examined me. Second, he reviewed the results on the spot. Third, he told me to schedule a biopsy for the same week.

I'd found large lumps before that *always* turned out to be non-cancerous cysts. Plus, having had two mammograms and an ultrasound within the year, I was more or less irritated to be going through the hassle. I doubted that I could work a biopsy into my schedule that week, or even that month, and told Dr. Auda that I would see what I could do. The roundtrip alone from my home to his office located south of Atlanta would consume three hours. I'd have to use up one of my precious few remaining vacation days. In response to my noncommittal attitude, he asked me to wait there a few minutes and disappeared.

When Dr. Auda returned, he presented a different option. If I could hang around another hour or so, he would perform the biopsy that day. I happily agreed because the day was already shot. It didn't occur to me that this prominent doctor had a good reason to accommodate my schedule. I was simply relieved that he salvaged a vacation day and saved me some gas money!

All of that replayed in my mind while I held for Dr. Auda, and trickles of concern began to saturate my thoughts. *Doctor Auda personally wants to speak to me?* Shit! This can't be good! It usually takes an act of congress to get a doctor on the phone.

"Hello, is this Lesa?" Doctor Auda asked in his grandfatherly tone.

"Yes, hi Dr. Auda," I answered.

"Lesa," he said with a slight hesitation (I imagined him scanning my records as he spoke), "we received the results back from your biopsy, and...ah...it's cancer. The tumor is malignant."

The rest of the conversation was a blur. I hung up with doctor Auda and called my parents.

Rugena, my mom, sweetly answered, "Hello?"

She is my confidante and trusted friend, the woman I most respect. She's sixty nine years old but I swear with her wrinkleless complexion, she could pass for fifty. She grew up in rural Georgia, the beautiful daughter of Hall County's prison warden. (In other words, young men knew that her daddy was armed!) Fortunately, the right fellow came along, and she and my dad Howard have been married for over fifty years. They lived in Frankfurt, Germany while he was stationed there in the army, and that's where my older brother Steve was born. Three years later, they moved back to Georgia, where they had me.

"Hello? Mom? Hey, it's me. Dr. Auda just called me. He said I have breast cancer."

A combination of shock, compassion, panic and urgency resonated in my mother's voice. She wanted to know every detail the doctor had discussed with me—from possible options to the scary unknowns.

When I hung up the phone, my mind was spinning. *I suppose I should tell my boss about this*, I thought. *This crap is probably going to involve a few days off work. Damn it! I wanted to use my vacation days to go to the beach.* (Remember, I said my mind was spinning—maybe that was a good thing.)

Still in a blur, I rose from my desk in slow motion and trudged down the long corridor to my boss's office. Once seated behind closed doors, I told her what I had just learned. She responded with compassion and understanding, which I appreciated, yet I caught a look in her expression that scared me at little. I almost felt like she could see into my future, and it wasn't pretty. Showing genuine support, she then insisted that I leave work early to discuss the matter with my family. Reluctantly, I accepted her suggestion. All in all, I was clueless about what my diagnosis entailed. No one close to me ever had breast cancer.

What should I do now? After arriving home, I didn't have time to think about it because my cell phone rang. "Hey there," he said. It was the sweet, familiar voice of Matt on the other end of the line. Matt and I had met a few months earlier. Things weren't so bad after all.

Two months earlier....

We met unexpectedly on a Friday night when my close friend Jamie and I were having dinner at a local Italian restaurant. Jamie and I had met years ago when she and I were teenagers. We lost touch for a while but fifteen years later, we ran into each other and formed a great lasting friendship.

While we waited to be seated, Jamie and I weaved our way through a plethora of people to the packed bar, which we scoped out for a couple seats. Since there weren't two seats together at the bar, we opted to stand in the crowded aisle. As we chatted, a boyishly handsome man seated at the bar turned towards us. Smiling, he politely interrupted our conversation.

"If you would like to sit, I'll move down one," he said.

I took the barstool next to him and Jamie sat beside me. Out of the corner of my eye, I caught him shifting his gaze back and forth from his menu to me. Of course, I spotted what he was up to because I was trying to get a better look at him. It was evident that he was younger than I, and *dang* handsome. I tried to seem nonchalant while Jamie and I ordered a couple coffees, checked our phone messages, and swapped stories about our day. When Jamie got a phone call, I busied myself by scanning the menu and sipping my coffee. However, my body language must have been speaking on my behalf because a conversation erupted between Dang Handsome and me.

We chatted politely about the menu and he enlightened me of his favorites. Distracted by his dark coffee brown eyes outlined with long lashes, his perfectly smooth complexion, and gorgeous white smile, I could barely concentrate on his words. Somehow, I listened well enough to learn that he was the middle child of first-generation Italian parents who lived in Pennsylvania. To my delight, he lived and worked just outside Atlanta. Tonight he was waiting on friends who were meeting him for dinner.

When our table was ready, Jamie followed the hostess. I waited for the check from the bartender. That's when Dang Handsome, a. k. a. Matt, took the opportunity to hand me his business card. He'd written his cell and home phone numbers on the back. He said to give him a call if I wanted to get together. Adrenaline shot straight through me. Yes, he was adorable, but I was having an anxiety attack over how young he looked. After I paid the bar tab, I smiled and handed his card back to him.

"How about we do this the other way around?" I said. "I'll give you my number and you can call me—if you like." That's the Southern girl in me. I gave him my number and walked away into the crowd to find Jamie.

Two nights later he called. We talked for three hours.

"Hi," I replied to the sweet familiar voice. I didn't plan to tell him about the cancer until I'd had time to digest the news myself, so we started off talking about nothing important. We were about to hang up when Matt said he'd call me back later during my drive home from work. I admitted that I wasn't at work, so, of course, he asked why. That's when I told him.

Five seconds of complete silence filled the airwaves before he spoke. "Are you ok?"

Obviously, by his tone, he was stunned. Sensing that he

was desperately searching for the right words, I felt a little sorry for him.

"Yeah, I'm fine. My boss made a big deal over it and insisted I leave work early."

"Well Lesa, it *is* a big deal," he said quietly.

Matt then revealed that his mother had breast cancer a few years prior, and his sister had tested positive for the hereditary gene; she too would likely have it one day. Again, he cautiously asked if I was *really* okay, and I repeated matter of factly that I was fine. I actually was fine at the moment. I had no idea what was about to happen… but Matt knew.

CHAPTER TWO

The Boyfriend

"One should never trust a woman who tells her real age. If she tells that, she'll tell anything." – Oscar Wilde

January

My first date with Matt was on a Thursday night. We planned for him to pick me up from my house, a Southern style, two-story with a large porch across the front. Around back, I have a pool and gazebo, which is where I was playing with my cocker spaniel, Rudy, until I heard Matt's car pull into the driveway. As I entered through the back with Rudy, Matt was knocking. I opened the front door to the beautiful smile I remembered so vividly from the restaurant.

I asked him in while I reached for my purse and coat. Meanwhile, Matt leaned down to pet Rudy. In return, Rudy licked him directly across the mouth. Awesome...my dog French kisses this man before I've even had a drink with him! At least he was a good sport about getting slobbered.

Matt suggested a trendy, eclectic restaurant only a few miles away. We were seated at a small, linen covered table. Jovial laughter rang out from the bar, which kept the atmosphere light as opposed to stuffy, but it actually wouldn't have mattered what was happening around us. Every so often our waiter's appearance would remind us that we were not alone because we were so absorbed in one another's every word. I studied his face and body language as he did mine. So far, I liked what I saw.

I learned that Matt, divorced for ten years, had no children. I told him that I too was divorced with a teenaged daughter. I joked about my being older than he was but he claimed he didn't think there was a big age difference and that he didn't care anyway.

Once back at my house, he pulled into my dimly lit driveway and parked. We continued our conversation, which had grown less formal, warmer. Finally, he leaned in and kissed me. Just as our lips parted, a bright light flicked across our faces. Simultaneously, we turned to see its source—the car headlights of my beautifully capricious daughter Alexandra wheeling into the driveway. Of course, my sixteen year old chose tonight of all nights to be on time! Matt turned back to me and looked me straight in the eyes. He said that kiss had not felt like any of his other first date kisses. I was tempted to ask if he was referring to the one with me or Rudy. Since he said he wanted to see me again the next night, I assumed he meant me.

I chose the restaurant on our second date. I was unbelievably nervous, but I was determined to relax and be myself. Yeah, right! If that were to happen, first of all, I'd be sitting in the restaurant in my gray, oversized drawstring sweats, ordering the most fattening thing the menu has to offer. Half my French manicure would be chipped off, and my legs wouldn't have been shaved in a week. Anyway, I digress….

During dinner Matt said he attended the University of Pennsylvania on an academic scholarship. Good, God! Could this date begin any worse? I already suspected he was Generations X, Y and Z younger than me, and now he's any Ivy Leaguer? Stop the madness! What's he going to think when he hears that the University of Georgia must have made a clerical mistake to have accepted me?

It was fun bantering back and forth about age, marriage, current events, age, the weather, age. He insisted that he wasn't as young as he looked and pulled out his driver's license and handed it across the table. *Oh, shit!* I was afraid to look, but I had to. Thirty-five it said. Oh no! I think I'm a *cougar!* In turn, I felt compelled to fess up. Hesitantly, I pulled my license from my purse and passed the laminated rectangle to him as if the information it contained was too devastating to articulate. I stared intently to read his expression. He gave my license a quick glance and handed it back while appearing completely unfazed.

Okay, I'm a realist. I tell him straight up, I'm well aware that handsome thirty-five-year-old men readily date twenty-something-year-olds. Looking directly at me with dark piercing eyes, he leaned across the table. With a smile playing on his lips, Matt said, "Oh, please, I'd be so bored."

I was forty-three.

Saturday, the next day, I was home doing laundry and thinking about my date with Matt when my cell rang. Speak of the devil! Since his Saturday night plans with the guys fell through, he wanted to know if I'd like to go out. That would make three nights in a row. Gee, I'm being pursued by a handsome, young, Ivy Leaguer. What shall I do?

"I'll be ready at eight," I told him.

From that point he began calling me on my way to work every morning, on my commute home in the afternoons, and later again in the evenings. He jokingly gave me a hard time for never calling him. I told him I was more comfortable with him calling me, but he challenged me to call him the next day. So I did. He joked that this was a big step for me. Honestly, I felt just a little crowded with all the calls at first. But I thought, no, he's sweet to me, I like him, and he seems genuinely to like me and of course there's that small detail that he's dang handsome. I quickly got over my need for space.

Soon thereafter Matt was cooking gourmet dinners for me at his home. He proved to be an awesome cook who was proud of his skills in the kitchen. My mouth watered just thinking about his scrumptious sautéed chicken grilled in Italian herbs and olive oil, topped with seasoned steamed broccoli and shrimp covered in a homemade béarnaise. I appreciated his culinary talents, but Matt's specialties sharply contrasted with my cooking. I was raised on Southern food. If my dinner's not fried, I need a shot glass chaser of cooking oil to get it down.

After dinner one night, we took his two collies, Bella and Ameika, for a walk through his upscale neighborhood. When we returned, we settled in for the night in front of the TV to eat dessert. Ameika jumped onto the couch with us, and her hefty paw landed directly on my left breast. It hurt, but I thought nothing more of it at the time. I had no idea the Collie had just stepped on my cancerous tumor.

Matt made her get off the couch, and we wrapped

ourselves tightly in a soft blanket. I was at ease being with Matt, kissing, talking and laughing in the dark. Even so, his sudden comment surprised me. Out of nowhere, he said, "I don't want to see anyone else but you."

His eyes never wavered from looking directly at the TV when he said it. Maybe he was unsure of what my expression might be and didn't want to look. In response, I slowly turned only my eyes to look at him. Our faces inches apart, he then turned his eyes directly to me and whispered, "I want to see where this is going to go with us."

I couldn't speak. I turned my gaze back to the TV. I desperately wanted to make sure that however I responded to him I meant it. The clock seemed to stop as I pondered an honest response. Finally, avoiding his eyes, I quietly replied, "I don't want to see anyone else either." I meant it. We sealed our decision with kisses tangled under a soft blanket. The collies slept peacefully at our feet.

From there, this new and unexpected beginning got even better. Whether at our favorite Mexican restaurant or searching for paint swatches for his basement project, we had fun together. At work during the day, he would send me text messages like XXXOOO and KISSES. I found an Internet site that translated English to Italian, so for fun I composed texts to him in Italian. It was amusingly apparent that this Italian boy was rusty with his Italian. Oh well, I was rusty in the cooking department.

The first time I cooked for Matt, I opted for a non-fried southern meal: chicken casserole, biscuits, and cranberry sauce. I was already nervous about the meal. To top it off, as I was taking the biscuits from the oven, Matt summoned my attention to the fact that Rudy had hopped up onto my dining room chair and was licking the butter dish. Here I was worried that my Southern cuisine and limited expertise in the kitchen wouldn't measure up. It never occurred to me that Rudy was going to turn the butter dish into an appetizer! Despite the real and imagined imperfections, Matt genuinely enjoyed the meal. As for my limited cooking skills, like my age, he didn't seem to care.

Unfortunately, our fun weekends of dining and drinks changed dramatically after I shared my diagnosis. Dinner conversation consisted of Matt plying me with questions about my PET scan and biopsy results, surgery dates, insurance, surgeons…everything. I saw concern in his face and I heard it in his voice.

Once, when we were on the phone together, we were talking about a tree in my yard that urgently needed to be cut. I laughed and said, "Eh, who cares, I may be buried under it next year!"

"That's not funny," he said quietly.

I laughed playfully.

"No! I mean it! That's not funny!" he snapped.

"Sorry." I replied. *(Note to self: One can lose ones sense of humor in times like these.)*

At two weeks before my mastectomy, with chemo to follow, I wondered what I should do about Matt. No, we had not dated for years, but there was something there between us. Was I really about to let this kind, young, handsome man stand by and watch as the chemo made me sick? As my hair fell out? As I became lethargic and anemic?

Out of the blue one day, my friend Jamie seemed to read my mind. "Lesa, I know you," she blurted. "I'll bet you're thinking of telling Matt you can't see him anymore because of the cancer, aren't you?"

She was right. Selfishly, I wanted him with me, but my conscience told me that it was only fair to let him go. What choice did I have?

CHAPTER THREE

Clueless

I have not yet begun to procrastinate.

April

I was dragging my feet about how to handle Matt. I called April, my friend since fifth grade. Even though we don't see one another very often because she lives in Florida, we talk frequently. I knew she would have some good advice.

As I dialed her number, I thought about the vacations we took together in years past. In my twenties, I worked as a flight attendant, and later in my thirties I was a corporate travel agent. Through my travel benefits, we had the opportunity to journey to elite destinations and stay at some of the top resorts in the Caribbean. Since April and I were both divorced, in the summer we'd hop a plane to one of the Lesser Antilles Islands.

On one of our trips, we stayed at a very luxurious resort on the Dutch side of the island of St. Maarten. Coincidentally, a regatta yacht race was coming to an end, and all the guys from the *Challenge America* yacht, who were also guests there, were having a cocktail party. We just so happened to stroll by the pool at the exact time their outdoor gala was underway. (Funny how that happened like that, huh?) Someone called to us, and in no time we had plans for the evening. An hour later we were attending their swanky caviar awards dinner as the invited guests of two gorgeous yachtsmen—identical twins, no less! At the table to my right sat Ted Turner Jr., Captain of *Challenge America* at that time, who was there with his wife. (There were two seats saved at the end of the table for Ted Sr. and his then wife Jane, but they never showed.) It was a fun, crazy party, and in the midst of drinking and dancing, Ted Jr. accidentally knocked his drink over in my dinner plate! It was late by then and I couldn't have cared less. We just looked at each other and burst out laughing. After dancing until 1:00am, the twins sneaked us past security on board *Challenge America*. April and I stood on board laughing and toasting champagne in the humid island breeze.

The next night a guy came knocking on our door in the middle of the night. I had met him earlier that day. He claimed to have lost his room key and was asking to stay with us for the night as he had no where to sleep except for the beach. Suspicious of this random guy, we didn't let him in. *What a loser to think we would fall for a line like that!* The next day we learned that he really did lose his key, and had to sleep on the beach. He also turned out to be a world renound photographer who had flown in to St Maarten especially to photograph the regatta race! *C'est la vie….*

Another summer we flew to Barbados and stayed in an elegant 19th century mansion that had been turned into a hotel that overlooked the coast. In addition to its breathtaking beach and gardens, the hotel grounds were home to small, wild monkeys that scampered freely about the place. Just down the road from our hotel was a casual bar where the locals hung out. April and I spent one evening there laughing and drinking until the wee hours of the morning. The next day we were told we'd been laughing it up with some celebrity athletes. We had no clue! Guess we need to watch a little more ESPN.

The next year was Jalousie Plantation in St Lucia. We stayed in a hillside villa surrounded by rainforest with breathtaking views of the Piton Mountains and the ocean. This is where we met Andrew. The young, tan, stunningly handsome Greek God lived in Manchester, England, yet spoke with an Australian accent. *(I thought I had died and gone to heaven.)* Working at the resort that summer, Andrew kind of became our personal guide shuttling us all over the property in his golf cart. To this day April claims I damn near knocked her down racing to get in the cart before her to sit next to him. (I claim that I don't recall what she's referring to, but I do have a scar on my right knee from it!)

Anyway, one afternoon Andrew took us by boat to a quaint little town on the island called Soufriere for a day of sightseeing and shopping. On our way back to the hotel, miles off the St Lucian coast, our boat ran out of gas. Andrew summoned help from a sweet local St Lucian man named Yo. Yo towed our huge boat all the way back to Jalousie with his little red canoe. It took forever to get back to the resort with only a canoe towing us, but we didn't care. Greek God. Accent. You understand.

After April and I had discussed my situation with Matt in depth, I jokingly asked, "So tell me….How does a girl date when her hair's falling out, she's missing a breast, and has two eyelashes?"

Without missing a beat, she replied as a question. "With the lights off?" Bitch thinks she's a comedian now! And I love her for it.

Point is, April and I have had many adventures together and I value her opinion.

Despite her optimism, I worried that Matt would have guilt if I stood by and he was forced to bring up the conversation of our parting ways. Jamie had already told me that she thought I should let the situation run its course naturally. Clueless as to how disruptive a mastectomy and chemo would be to my life, I opted for a temporary solution. I would postpone any discussion about Matt and me not seeing each other anymore until after the operation. At some point before I started chemo, I would initiate a heart-to-heart that gave Matt a guilt-free "out."

I won't deny that I *did not* want to have this impending conversation. At the same time, I wanted to do the right thing for him.

Leading up to the surgery, Matt expressed his desire to do something for me—anything! He offered to help with yard work—trimming hedges, cutting my grass. I wouldn't let him. I didn't want to appear needy. When he cooked dinner for me at his house, he started sending the leftovers home with me. This I accepted. His meals were delicious, and if he *needed* to do something for me, I felt cooking was a fair option. For all his other offers, I thanked Matt for asking but always declined his help.

One Saturday he called to say he was on the road to my house to cut my grass. He had his mower loaded on back of his truck and wouldn't take no for an answer. Matt sweated in the hot sun for four straight hours in my yard that day cutting, raking and hauling grass, refusing to let me lift a finger except to bring him water and watch after his collies. When he was done, exhausted and covered with grass, he sat down next to me on my driveway. We talked for a few minutes, and I realized he was really scared for me. He looked at me differently now.

The next thing I knew, Matt said that he was taking three days off work the week after my surgery. I thought he meant for some remodeling he was doing in his house. He explained the time was for *me*. Assuming my family would be with me immediately after the surgery, he would be available the following week just in case I needed him. I was touched beyond words. Remembering that my daughter Alex raved about his homemade meatballs, Matt added that he would be making spaghetti and meatballs, too, when I got home from the hospital.

With two days before my surgery, Matt had asked me to come by his house after work. Sitting on his kitchen counter were the ingredients for the homemade spaghetti sauce he'd promised. I deeply appreciated his efforts. At the same time, I felt guilty for screwing up everything with the cancer.

The next day at work, my phone vibrated with a text message from Matt. "*KISSES… me,*" he wrote. That night, with my surgery in the morning, he called to tell me not to worry. He'd give me a big kiss when I get home.

CHAPTER FOUR

Overwhelmed

"It's not that I'm afraid to die. I just don't want to be there when it happens." —Woody Allen

Pure unadulterated hell on earth best described the one night my insurance company kindly paid for me to stay in the hospital after the mastectomy. One of the nurses said I was "lucky" that my insurance company paid for one night. Many women, she said, are forced to go home the same night as their operations.

After surgery, someone rolled me down a long hallway to my room. I have a foggy memory of my mother being in the room, and my father and brother standing in the doorway with worried, forced smiles on their faces. My mother stayed with me through the night. As she watched closely over me, she noticed a red rash suddenly appear on the side of my face. Within minutes it covered my entire face.

My mother was told that I was given Benadryl for the rash, and it *seemed* to work. Although the rash began to fade, shortly after, my mother noticed that my breaths seemed fewer and farther between one another. Over a period of a few minutes, they grew significantly less frequent. Something had gone wrong. She tried to wake me and couldn't. I was unconscious. She ran into the hallway and down to the nurse's station for help. I almost stopped breathing altogether.

A nurse immediately called in the hospital's respiratory unit. I'm not sure how long I was out, but when I came to, the room was full of medical personnel running about. The reason I finally came to? They cut my morphine off—completely. Holy shit!!!

Let me be extremely clear here: You *never* want to be without morphine when you've just had your breast amputated and an eight-inch cut from the center of your back to underneath your arm where skin's been grafted and muscle moved around to the breast area. This added procedure is called a latissimus flap that uses muscle and skin from your upper back to create a new breast mound after a mastectomy. It was two surgeries in one! One doctor performed the mastectomy, and then a second surgeon stepped in to perform the reconstructive latissimus flap. I felt like I had been sawed in half! With nothing for pain, I was hanging over the bed rail reaching out to and pleading for anyone who'd listen for drugs.

In response, they continued scurrying around my room talking amongst themselves. It was another fifteen or twenty minutes that may as well have been days before they came to the conclusion that I couldn't have any more morphine, but I could have an alternative pain medication in pill form that would take what seemed like an eternity to enter my system. This was the most agonizing, painful night on record in my memory.

Later, when I relayed what happened to one of my doctors unrelated to the surgery, he said it sounded like I had been overdosed with morphine. I believe if my mother hadn't been by my bed watching me so closely, I could have died.

Matt asked me if my mother would phone him from the hospital after the surgery for an update. When Mom made the call, I also spoke with him briefly.

Unexpectedly, my ex-husband, Alexandra's Dad, came to see me at the hospital. His visit was touching for many reasons. For one, the hospital was more than fifty miles away, so it wasn't as if he just dropped by. He also came with gifts specially chosen because he knew I would appreciate them—one dozen red roses, chocolates, and a black and white sketch by a local artist. I showed my gratitude by puking every ten minutes the entire time he was there. He helped out by retrieving fresh containers for me to hurl in.

I went home the day before Easter, and Matt said he wanted to see me Easter night if that was okay with me. I said sure even though I looked like a train wreck and felt like pure hell. I was carved up like a Christmas turkey with three drains hanging out of me and hundreds of stitches in my chest and back. All the while, I was trying to decide which of my silk PJs would be most flattering to a bandaged torso. (My navy pair seemed to bring out the dark circles under my eyes rather nicely!)

I was overwhelmed; my body, brain and spirit were in shock. Taking a shower was a two-hour event. I cut arm holes in a rain cape to cover my bandaged chest and the bandaged incision across my back so they wouldn't get wet. I couldn't raise one arm at all, and the other one wouldn't go much farther than my ear. Oh, and I still had to contend with the three drains coming out of me. Thankfully, Mom helped me with showers and maneuvering in and out of bed for the first week I was home. Getting dressed was a major task in itself because every slight movement hurt even with pain medication. I couldn't even sit up without help.

I was waiting for Matt to arrive Easter night, but nine o'clock came and went and he hadn't arrived. It was time to drain fluid from those stupid drains. I wanted to wait until he had come and gone, but I had to measure and record the amount of fluid accumulated in them for the doctor. By ten o'clock there was still no Matt, and he hadn't called. Wearily, I called it a night, and Mom helped me with the drains and into bed.

The lingering effects of the anesthesia and morphine, and the enormity of the diagnosis itself were all taking their toll on me mentally. I couldn't sleep, and when I did, I had horrendous nightmares. It was difficult to think clearly and my body ached. With everything, I was distressed and confused by what Matt had done.

The next day Matt made apologies as to why he didn't come or call, but then I didn't hear from him for days. That is when I decided to call and leave him a heartfelt message (yes, me who never calls him) that if he had decided not to see me anymore it was okay. I told him I accept whatever he was trying to do and to not to be afraid to call me back— even if that was the case.

Five days later, Matt called. He said after fifteen years with his employer, his job had been eliminated along with a few hundred others. He was extremely upset and bitter. He assured me that the breakdown in communication between us occurred because he had flown to his company's corporate headquarters in Texas on the spur of the moment with some colleagues in an attempt to save their jobs. He said he had sent me a text about what was going on with him, but I never received it. He went on to say that he got my message left on his voicemail, and added that he was sorry I had misunderstood his actions by thinking he didn't want to see me anymore. When I said it was all okay, he quietly responded, "No, it's not ok," as though he felt badly for the miscommunication.

He asked me how I was feeling. "I'm fine," I answered nonchalantly.

"You're not fine," he whispered.

Before we hung up, he conveyed all was good between us.

Matt never contacted me again after that day. I have not seen him since.

His timing bordered on cruel. It'd been five days since I arrived home from the hospital; I was on mental overload from the brutal physical nature of the surgery. My mind was blurry from the side effects of the anesthesia and the stress of knowing I had to be back at work in four days. The fact that Matt went away was not what disturbed me the most. What bothered me was *how* I was blindsided by his lack of character in which he went about it.

May

My boss and I were scheduled to attend a conference for work in Orlando that had been on the calendar for months. I didn't want to look helpless, so I told her I could still make the trip. A young coworker from our marketing department with whom I worked with to set up the trip stopped by my office one afternoon. She offered to attend the conference for me if I was not able. I didn't know her extremely well, which made her gesture all the more touching. For her to go in my place was in no way self-serving. She was simply a compassionate human being reaching out to help. I declined her offer, but what a classy girl.

For the trip I had arranged to be picked up by an airport shuttle. It never occurred to me that the shuttle ride would beat the hell out of me. The driver darted in and out of lanes at ninety miles per hour through Atlanta traffic. Although everyone on board was holding on with white knuckles, we all continued to bump into each other. It had only been thirty days since the surgery, and all the jarring and bumping on the forty-minute ride pulled on my incisions and was killing me.

Thankfully, the flight to Orlando was fine, however; when I arrived at the hotel, representatives were handing out satchels of workbook materials to the conference participants that weighed about fifteen pounds, and I was supposed to lift no more than ten. It hurt like hell to carry the bag, but I didn't want to impose upon my boss for help. I rode the elevator up to my floor, and when I knew no one was looking, I dropped the satchel and hooked the shoulder strap around my ankle. In heels, I dragged the bag with my foot all the way to my room and kicked it in the door.

That night, after working my company's booth until ten pm, I crawled in bed with wounds throbbing. I was too exhausted to cry. I vaguely remember feeling tears stream down the side of my face to the pillow, but only for a second, and I was out until morning. I arrived back home in Atlanta from Orlando on Thursday night. Friday morning was my first chemo.

I would get a round of chemo every three weeks until six rounds had been completed. When over, I'd continue to get an IV of a drug called Herceptin—a type of gene therapy drug—every three weeks until I have one year's worth in my system. Herceptin is given to some cancer patients who are HER2Nu positive. It stands for "Human Epidermal growth factor Receptor 2" and is a protein giving higher aggressiveness in breast cancers. It is a lot like taking the chemo except it wouldn't make me sick or my hair fall out.

The scariest part of chemo would be the unknown. The horrific side effects you've heard about and not knowing what will happen to you or when can really screw with your mind. Imagine if someone said there was a room full of people swinging baseball bats as hard as they could. Now you must go into the room blindfolded and walk around in there for five months. You wouldn't see it coming, but you'll get hit…repeatedly. That's how I imagined chemo would be. I was right.

Doctor Auda told me my cancer had a high chance of reoccurrence. How fast breast cancer cells grow is rated on a scale from one to three. Disorganized, irregular growth patterns in which many cells are in the process of making new cells is grade three with a less favorable outcome. My cancer was grade three, the fastest growing type. The tumor they removed from my chest had nearly doubled in size between the time it was discovered and the surgery three weeks later.

I agonized that I would undergo the mastectomy, have

all the chemo treatments and the reconstructive surgery, and that the cancer would come back and kill me anyway. Either that or I'd be in and out of hospitals with cancer from now until I became an old woman. Those thoughts were overwhelmingly depressing.

Not only that, I was reading the fine print on a mile-high stack of paperwork from the oncologist when I located a passage that stated the chemo I was taking could cause Leukemia. I asked my oncologist if this was true for me. He said yes, that was true, but if I got it, it would likely not be for another twenty-five years. Not really the warm and fuzzy answer I was hoping for.

CHAPTER FIVE

Beautiful Strangers

*"Kind words can be short and easy to speak,
but their echoes are truly endless."*
— Mother Teresa

I was in awe of the outpouring of kindness from coworkers who learned about my cancer. One group collectively gave me a huge wicker gift basket filled with lotions, PJs, caps, health foods, dark chocolate, and an assortment of other items. The card attached to the basket contained money to go towards the purchase of a wig.

One day when I arrived at work early in the morning, I found flowers waiting at my office door. One lady gave me a silver bracelet with a pink ribbon charm attached that had belonged to a family member of hers who had fought breast cancer. Co-workers, some I hardly knew at the time, would stop by my office door, ask how I was and share personal stories with me.

Mike was one who stopped by on occasion to talk. His young daughter-in-law had been fighting cancer for a few years and was on chemo. He would come in my office and sit for a few minutes, ask how I was feeling and I'd ask how his daughter-in- law was doing. When he hadn't stopped by in a while, I assumed he'd been busy with work. When I spotted him one day in the hall, I asked about his daughter-in-law. Mike told me she had died. He had stayed away because he couldn't bear to tell me. Our conversations and experiences bonded us. A few months later he invited me to accompany him, his wife and family to a breast cancer walk in Atlanta. Together we all walked and my heart went out to this family for their loss.

Sherry was another co-worker and personal friend who'd stop at my office door briefly each day. One afternoon she asked if she could come in and close the door.

"Sure." I answered, puzzled but intrigued.

She shut the door and sat down.

"Can I pray *with* you?" she asked.

"Yes," I answered.

Sherry slid her chair towards mine. Then she reached and touched my hand, bowed her head and began to pray. Her words were unwaveringly poignant. Bowing my head and fighting back tears, I opened my eyes and looked at Sherry. I watched her speak to God on my behalf. I did not see a co-worker; I saw an extraordinary beautiful soul.

Cancer survivors within my company, some I had not previously met, heard about my breast cancer and inquired if they could stop by to see me. They came to me offering moral support, advice, and sometimes sharing personal stories with me. Not just once but many times. These beautiful strangers became my friends.

I could go on about numerous others who took time out of their day for me. Words can't express how much each meant to me. To those of you who shared your stories and lives with me, thank you. You made me feel less alone. You helped put my broken spirit back together again.

When I arrived home that night with the gift basket, I was so excited to show it to Alex and look at each item again. But Alex wasn't home, as she had gone to the movies with a friend. Later into the evening she called me. She had seen Matt in line at the movie theatre near our home. Admittedly, she had been hesitant to mention it to me. I assured her I was fine with the fact that she had told me. I was curious, however, if Matt had seen her. She said yes, they made eye contact, and then he looked straight down at the floor.

Whatever—jerk still owes us meatballs!

Patient: "Doctor, my hair keeps falling out. Have you got anything to keep it in?"
Doctor: "What about a cardboard box?"

June

Alex turned seventeen years old on June 8th. A week later my hair started coming out in handfuls. In the days leading up to it, the roots of my hair were especially sore. It actually hurt to comb, brush or move my hair around in any way so I decided to shave my head. Who wants to worry about leaving a trail of hair down the hall at work?

Alex went with me to a hair salon. When I explained what I needed done, a woman led us to a private area in the back. As she began shaving my head, I watched clumps of hair falling to the floor making me feel like I was disappearing as well. Redirecting my attention, I listened as she talked. She said that she was from a big family, one of six sisters, and they all had to have hysterectomies at some point in their lives. Each of them had the opportunity to have children...except for her. She was twenty-eight years old when she had to have her hysterectomy and never had the chance to have children. I could see in her eyes that she had really wanted them. She seemed sad. As I listened, I looked down at my long blonde locks on the dusty floor then up into the mirror and saw the reflection of my bald head... and more importantly, my daughter beside me holding my hand. I was the lucky one here.

Before Alex and I left the salon that day, we thanked the woman and I hugged her. She refused to let me pay her one cent.

On Monday morning I wore a blonde wig to work. I realize I have bigger worries, but wearing a wig for the first time in front of friends and coworkers with a bald head lurking underneath was brutal on the psyche. I felt old, weak, insecure and artificial.

On Wednesday my boss and I were scheduled to give a presentation for thirty or so people, who included VPs and the president of the company. Standing before them was torture. Still foggy from the chemo, it was extremely hard to concentrate, but I was desperately trying to hide it. On top of everything, during the meeting, someone remarked that maybe my position should be eliminated if no one knew or understood the benefit of my job. In reaction to the comment, my head kind of tilted forward, my eyebrow arched to my fake hair line and I didn't realize my mouth was open. This quirky look on my face made the entire room break out into good natured laugher. They thought I had a great sense of humor about the comment, but actually what was going through my mind was what a cherry on the cake it would be to lose my job and insurance while my chemo alone was over $5000 every three weeks. That's not to mention surgeries and hospital stays!

Kyle, a VP from Florida, stopped by my office afterwards. Knowing I was on chemo, he wanted to reassure me that the remark someone had made about my job was only figure of speech. I had long ago determined that he was a good guy. We had met just one month after I joined the company at a corporate dinner. Although I appreciated his attempt to calm me, I only hoped he was right.

This week did not get any better. Three days later, I fell down a flight of stairs at home. I was wearing a pair of those soft, plushy, fluffy house socks with slick bottoms. The State of Georgia should require a waiting period like the one required for purchasing a gun before someone can own a pair of those damn things. Words of advice: Don't hurry down a flight of stairs wearing them after a mastectomy. My foot slipped off the top step and sent me flying through the air like an Olympic gymnast. I automatically tried to catch myself on the way down, but the wall caught my left arm and bent it backwards. I imagined every stitch ripping out of my chest and back. My other arm struck a few rail posts on the opposite side of the stairs while my butt smacked the edge of two steps. Finally, my knees and head collided with the hardwood floor at the bottom. I lay stunned and motionless in the dark.

In addition to those hazardous socks, fashioned in neon green, my drawstring pajama pants were donned with red and white candy canes. The comfy faded blue shirt I was wearing was so old that I couldn't remember if I wore it in middle school, or used to dust with it. This fashion statement was all topped off with a knit pink stocking cap to cover my perpetually cold, bald head. The fall, which made me feel like a feeble old woman, hurt as much mentally as physically. While I blindly felt around the floor for my glasses, Rudy rushed to my side to lick the tears off my face. The aroma of his Beefy Bites breath added insult to injury, and then before I knew it, he had swept his tongue right into my mouth. I wasn't sure whether to worry more about the germs on my weakened immune system or since I hadn't been kissed in a while that I was a little turned on by it!

Slowly, I pulled myself up. Rudy followed me into my bathroom and watched while I drew a hot bath. After I got in, Rudy sat loyally on the edge of the tub and took an occasional drink of the warm water. He looked at me with sad cocker eyes, as though he wished he could help. He did.

CHAPTER SIX

Midst Of Chaos

I'm so far behind I thought I was first.

My *!#%@!* pea green swimming pool is stressing me out. I had professionals open it for me, but the water remained green two weeks later. I spent a truckload of money on pool chemicals, but the color still wasn't close to blue. Turns out this happens when sand in the pump hasn't been changed in a number of years. Shit! The job was going to cost me two hundred dollars. I just spent two hundred dollars on routine maintenance.

Adding to my stress, I had to leave work on chemo treatment days two hours early to make my appointment. After treatment, I often went directly to the grocery store on the way home. Anyone passing me in the dark parking lot while I'm loading my groceries in the trunk would quickly look away. I know they wondered why I was crying. If you've ever lifted an oversized bag of dog food in the rain after chemo while healing from a mastectomy, you'd understand.

Never mind that I was stripped of energy from the work day.

After loading the car, I headed home, unloaded the groceries, let Rudy out, opened the mail, sorted through the bills, and worked on pool problems. This usually involved sticking my hand, still blue from the IV hours prior, in the green pool to unscrew a clogged jet or empty a skimmer basket full of leaves, frogs, lizards, and sometimes a snake or two. Later, I paid the bills, fed Rudy and our cat Diamond, started a load of laundry, and took out the trash. On weekends there were weeds to pull, leaves to rake, and bushes to cut. Thank God Dad cut my grass and Mom trimmed the shrubs, even though I told them not to bother. I had too many things to remember to do and I was in a daze from the chemo brain fog.

Among my to-do list was remembering to *always* close the toilet seat lid. The oncology nurse said that chemo in my urine could remain in the water even after flushing. Rudy liked to have a nice cool drink of toilet bowl water from time to time, and the potent chemicals might harm him. Great! I've got *lethal urine*. Maybe Mel Gibson will play me in the movie.

My chemo dosage was extremely strong. My doctor let me in on this fact, but I had already figured that out. A woman at my oncologist office had cancer spread throughout her body and was on the exact same chemo treatment as me. It knocked her into the hospital after her first dose, and then later she arrived for her next appointment in a wheelchair. To be safe, Alex slept in the bed with me or next to me on the couch the first night after each new round of chemo in case I had a major complication.

Although the chemo continued to cloud my thoughts, I tried to conceal it at work. I sat at my desk struggling to concentrate on tasks and conversations. I reread incoming emails and outgoing replies five times just to make sure I had my facts straight.

Also, the chemo made my surgery incisions burn like someone was holding a match to them which was distracting as well. Coworkers would tell me how good I looked on days when it was all I could do to sit upright in my chair. It didn't help that the tight elastic inside my dumb ass wig gave me a pounding headache every single day. Also disconcerting was a strange faint beeping sound I often heard coming from behind me.

I looked for the positive elements around me, but every day I could hear the news coming from the TV just outside my office in the break room. It was continuous coverage of World Wars, tragedy, death and even the bird flu. Not exactly the highlight of my day to be marinating in chemo while hearing reports of a possible bird flu outbreak in town.

"Never loan your car to anyone to whom you've given birth." - Erma Bombeck

I'd been on chemo one month when I received a call that Alex had been in a car wreck. Just out of the shower, I grabbed any clothes I could find and rushed out the door. The first thing I saw upon arriving at the scene was her smashed silver Pontiac Sunfire in pieces from one side of the road to the other. My heart jumped out my chest until

I spotted Alex standing in the midst of the chaos. Our eyes met and I realized she was fine. I took a breath.

Three other vehicles were involved, but somehow everyone walked away without a scratch. I was immensely relieved that no one involved was hurt. Even so, Alex was ticketed as the at-fault driver. Also, with our car totaled, she had no transportation to school. Her senior year started in two weeks.

I spent every lunch hour on the phone with some combination of the following: the car insurance company, the tow yard, a rental car company. Otherwise, I was looking for another car for Alex. Fortunately, I had full coverage on the car. If not dealing with car issues, I was juggling my doctor appointments.

About a week after the accident, while still in the middle of cleaning up problems, I drove straight home from work. All I could think about was sitting down in front of the TV with my dinner to forget all this shit for a little while. I was almost there—just having plopped down on the sofa and flicked on the TV—at last taking a deep breath. *Ahhh!* Exhausted but finally settled, I picked up my fork to take the first bite when I heard a loud *click.* The TV went black and the lights went out. For a moment, I sat in complete darkness. (A power outage hit the area.) Let's just say I screamed a few things at God that I later told him I was sorry for.

On Sunday, my parents invited my brother Steve, his wife Donna, my niece Kenzie, and Alex and me over for lunch. No one in my family except Alex had seen me since I had shaved my head. After lunch my wig was making my head throb as usual, so I asked who wanted to see my bald freak show head. Every hand in the room went up. I stood in the center of the room and removed my wig. In unison, everyone began assuring me how bad I did NOT look.

"Well Lesa," Mom said, "you've got a very pretty shaped head."

Thanks Mom. I always have wanted an attractive skull!

Dad told me to go upstairs and pick out any baseball cap from his collection that I wanted. I'd never before had people try to make me feel good about looking ugly. It was surreal. Until chemo, I'd considered myself reasonably attractive. I was Miss Sophomore in 1977, for God sakes, and now I have a pretty shaped head? That afternoon, I crossed the threshold into the twilight zone.

Every day on my drive to and from work, I played one song over and over again. Listening to "I Can Only Imagine" was the only thing that temporarily relieved my fear of dying. I've believed in God, Jesus, heaven and hell all my life, but I'm here to tell you the thought of dying, not being here on planet Earth, where everyone I know existed, paralyzed me with fear. This song is about someone wondering what he will do when he sees God in heaven for the first time. Will he stand in his presence or will he fall to his knees in awe? I wondered what I would do as well.

Somehow, the words made dying seem less terrifying, but I was still scared and extremely sad. My doctor's office staff noticed and offered me depression medication. I refused it. Life as it had been for me was gone, and I wanted to deal with the multitude of demons in my head on my own terms.

Seeing what other people were going through at my

oncologist office forced me to examine my own possibility of dying. One day while I sat waiting to be called in, I heard a very loud thud that resonated throughout the building. I knew a human being had just hit the floor. As all the nurses went running to see, I slowly peered with one eye around the corner.

There lying on floor in the main hallway, a burly looking man was groaning. He had just left the chemo room and was heading down the hall to leave when he landed face first on the floor. His face was bleeding and he wasn't moving. The only sound he made was a hair-raising groan. The doctor and nurses worked diligently to help him, to no avail. Paramedics whisked in and loaded him onto a stretcher. They all disappeared out the door to the hospital across the street.

It was chilling to see this big, strong man so helpless and fragile.

As I retreated back to my little chair in the waiting room, my elbow knocked over a small holder of pamphlets sitting on the table next to me. As I picked them up and placed them back into the holder, I read the front: "HOSPICE CARE." *Good grief!* (No pun intended.) I could do with a little more inspiring reading material around here. What else am I going to find, a magazine advertising burial plots? Ugh!

July

Today, sitting in a recliner in the chemo room, I looked around, taking in the scenery, as the medicine flowed into me. Gray recliners lined the walls. Standing next to each chair was a tall, portable chemo-dispensing machine.

Periodically, a machine would beep, prompting a nurse to walk over, press some buttons and then retreat back to her station. To remind us of the normal world outside those walls, two televisions were mounted to the ceiling on either side of the room.

During that suspended time period, my cell rang. Alex was calling to discuss the details of her planned whereabouts that night and her curfew. I told her to unload the dishwasher, move the wet clothes from the washer to the dryer, and let Rudy out before she left. When I hung up, I overheard a woman sitting nearby tell someone that her job was about to be posted because she'd missed too many days of work.

Next to me a woman talking on her cell was telling one of her kids why it wasn't possible to go over to the neighbor's house to play. Her name was Cindy. She was a school teacher with two young children. Like me, she was a single mom with breast cancer. Appearing to be in her early thirties, Cindy's big green eyes and quick smile matched her bubbly, full-of-life personality. From talking with her, I learned that she had a lumpectomy, the cancer returned, so she had to undergo a mastectomy as well.

When tested, Cindy had thirty-one positive lymph nodes, meaning that was the number which contained cancer cells. The higher the number, the more aggressive some doctors believe a person's cancer to be.

Although she was currently finished with chemo, Cindy continued to take Herceptin as she was HER2nu positive like me. She told me after one of her radiation treatments some spots showed up on the inside middle of her chest. The spots turned out to be cancer in her skin. She said one of her doctors commented that it was strange that the spots appeared on the opposite side of her breast from where her tumor had been. She told me she thought she knew what happened.

Before Cindy's mastectomy, she had large breasts. During the surgical removal of her tumor, the surgeon lapped some extra skin over to the center of her chest then sewed her up. She felt this explained why the spots showed up there. With a sense of humor, she went on to say that with everything going on in her life, her boyfriend asked to borrow money! The entire room burst into laughter. We had no idea anyone else was listening. Even people who were lying motionless, seemingly off in another place, chuckled. Of course, Cindy added, the guy soon disappeared.

Well, what do you know? I found a friend with the same good taste in men as *me*!

A few weeks later, I ran into Cindy again in the chemo room.

"Hi", she said in her usual cheerful voice. She sat in the recliner next to me.

"Oh, wow, your nails look beautiful!" I commented.

She smiled at me and looked down to admire her gorgeous, acrylic French manicured nails. "Yeah, it's kind of all I've got right now, you know?"

I returned her smile and nodded. I knew what she meant. We had scars under our clothes, no hair, no eyelashes, few eyebrows, pale skin, and sinking veins in our arms. Our own natural nails were weakened from the chemo, and tended to peel off like tape. Having our nails done helped us feel a little bit pretty. In a few minutes, the nurse came over and adjusted Cindy's IV. When she went back to the nurses' station, Cindy leaned over to me. Touching the front right side of her head, she asked, "Can you tell my hair is coming out again right here?"

I could tell, but I replied, "No, no, not at all. You look great."

She leaned closer. Looking me in the eye, she whispered, "The cancer spread to my brain. I've got to start chemo all over again."

I'll never forget the look we exchanged in that moment. No words describe it. I tried to comfort her with the most encouraging words I had in me. But we both knew. I never saw Cindy again after that day. Nurses told me she died not long after.

Still July

I was burned-out from staying in during my lunch hour most days to handle personal issues, so I decided to go out to pick up food and bring it back to my office. Out of the blue, while waiting at a nearby restaurant for my to-go order, I felt a sharp, extremely intense, stabbing pain in my chest. It was so sudden and hurt so badly that I gasp out loud and grabbed my chest. The killer sensation happened again and again. I thought I was having a heart attack.

After my outburst, people were staring, and a restaurant employee approached to ask if I was okay. Fighting back tears while still bent over clutching my chest, I looked up at her and whispered, "I don't know."

The stabbing pain continued for about five minutes then ceased. I paid for my food and hurried to my car. I drove back to my office. Still shaking, I called my doctor's office. The nurse told me this happens to some people during treatment. It meant only that one of the powerful shots they had given me was working.

I hung up and slumped weakly on my desk. You'd think they'd give you a heads up that the teeny little shot they gave you may have side effects comparable to a butcher knife being thrust into your chest! I looked at the clock on my computer—four more hours to go in the work day.

CHAPTER SEVEN

Freak Show

"I never forget a face, but in your case I'll be glad to make an exception."
—Groucho Marx

Some breast cancer patients will have a port put in their chest to receive chemo treatments. My doctor requested that I get one. I didn't want a port, so I asked him if there was any way around it. He explained that I could take the chemo in my arm or hand as long as no complications arose.

As a result, the back of my right hand at the point where the IV entered was perpetually blue, sometimes from a blown vein. A blown vein (or tear) resulted at times when a nurse stuck a needle in the top of my hand to take blood or insert an IV. With bleeding under the skin, the area sometimes blew up to the size of a golf ball. Although each one eventually went away, a blown vein hurt for days.

From two months of needles, I had a sore blue and yellow hand. My right arm screamed "drug addict" because the chemo caused the veins to collapse, and red streaks ran from the bend in my arm to my wrist. Typically, I wore long sleeved shirts with long floppy cuffs at work to hide the tops of my hands.

I was anemic too, so my complexion was white as a sheet with the exception of dark circles under my eyes. Making matters worse, I could not sleep more than three hours per night. So much for beauty rest! I was desperate for sleep and not having it made my work days worse. One of my doctors prescribed Ambien sleeping pills. I'd never taken any kind of sleeping pill before, so I was wary of side effects. These things are very powerful, but they work.

Alert enough to care how I looked, I bought under-eye concealer by the bucket load and applied darker face makeup to give my chalky skin some color. As my hair loss progressed, I had to color in about fifty percent of my brows, and the extra mascara I caked on basically made my two eyelashes look like four. A blond wig topped off this montage of facial artwork. I got up at six am for work every morning just to turn myself into this freak show.

I remained in a daze with foggy thoughts and overwhelming fatigue. And what is that beeping noise?

Over the weekend, Emily, my friend Ellen's daughter, wanted me to take her engagement photographs. Photography's my hobby, and word-of-mouth requests come every so often. Ellen had prearranged for the pictures to be taken at her friend's home, which was absolutely breathtaking. The property included a rock swimming pool and fish pond, an enormous circular water fountain, a lush flower garden, a glistening lake with ducks, and horses in the distance. I took about 80 photographs of Emily and her fiancé Kenny and later edited and burned the images to a disk and gave the disk to Emily.

When Emily took the disk to Wal-Mart to have prints made, the salespeople told her that they couldn't reproduce professional photos without a copyright release. Frustrated, she called me at work. Emily wanted some of the pictures for a party that same night. The runaround Wal-Mart gave Emily annoyed her, but I couldn't have been more flattered. My photographs were deemed to be professional!

In the coming weeks, I planned to attend their elegant outside wedding, which overlooked a large gorgeous lake. I had looked forward to the event, but I dreaded going anywhere in my stupid wig. Wearing it made me self-conscious. Besides, I'd see people there who I hadn't seen in ages.

Even so, Alex and I went together. We parked our car and then headed down a long, winding pathway that lead to the entrance. With each step, all I could think about is that I am an absolute freak show in this wig and God, please don't let it be windy today. I didn't think that Emily and Kenny would be amused if their cherished wedding ceremony video captured a blonde wig flying past their pastor's head.

Distracted and anxious, I'd been looking down as we walked towards the gate to the property. Lifting my head, I came face-to-face with an expansive, elegantly framed, black-and-white photograph of Emily and Kenny. Facing each other, Kenny was kissing Emily on the forehead. It was one of the photographs I had taken. I didn't think about that wig the rest of the day!

Later in July

I finally found a replacement car for Alex, coincidentally, the same make, model and color as the one she wrecked. It differed in that the new car was a two-door instead of a four-door, and this model displayed the added feature of a sunroof. I had made arrangements to purchase and pick up the car after work with the stipulation that the car dealership fix two problems. The sales manager assured me the work was completed and the car was ready.

As usual, I'd run out of energy at work by two o'clock that day, but I still had to drive two hours to the dealership when I got off at five. Both of my parents came with me so someone could drive the new car home. Upon arriving, however, I immediately saw that one of my requested repairs remained undone. I then learned that the other problem was not corrected.

My pulse rate was off the charts as I entered the car dealership to meet my salesman. When he claimed that the dealership had, in fact, taken care of the issues, the man was lucky that I did not have enough strength to kick. Instead, I walked him to the car and touched the physical evidence. In response, he told me that the department in charge of such matters must have missed it, and unfortunately, all of said mechanics had gone home for the night. With that, he just stood there and looked at me. That was it!

I requested to speak to his boss and his boss's boss. Each one jerked me around. Oh, those poor arrogant men had no idea they were crossing a wrung out, sick bitch in a blonde wig running on pure exhaustion with poison in her veins. A four-hour standoff ensued that night with me standing toe-to-toe with four condescending car salesmen.

I would have dropped dead on their dusty car dealership floor before letting them take advantage of me. To sum up, I drove home *that night* with my newly purchased car, *all* of my requests resolved by the dealership, and a hint of a weary smile lurking beneath my blonde wig.

August

The chemo was kicking my butt. I had the worst day and night from hell of nonstop vomiting, diarrhea, aching bones, muscles, back, legs, arms and face. I took one vacation day and was back at work the next morning. I sat at my desk so weak that day thinking that if God let me die right here on my desk calendar, it would be a relief. Probably because I felt so bad, my mind kept going over how I got in this mess to begin with.

How come my mammograms didn't spot the cancer earlier? My oncologist told me that judging by the size and type of my tumor, it had to have been in me for seven or eight years. *What?!!*

Apparently, mammograms overlook a high percent of breast cancers. My oncologist told me this like it was common knowledge, accepted. People like me will either die because it's been overlooked too long, or the doctors start working on it late in the game and patients suffer longer with chemo and sometimes still end up dying. Meanwhile, if women had annual MRIs, many cancers could possibly be found sooner and perhaps result in little or no need for chemo. If a mammogram had found my cancer earlier, the chances are that I could have avoided chemotherapy.

Slumped over my desk, I pondered why the Hubble Telescope could see fungus on Jupiter twelve billion light years away, yet the mammograms we relied on to detect breast cancer had trouble seeing through a few layers of human flesh. I might as well have had a Polaroid taken of my breast for all the good it did me!

Again, what the heck was that beeping sound? It wasn't constant, but every so often during the day I distinctly heard the noise, which seemed to be directly behind my ear. I was certain that it originated from something in my office. I checked my computer and printer, but no machines in my office were beeping. Chemo had to be playing tricks. Strangely, the beeping sounded just like the machine that was by my bed at the hospital when I woke up from my mastectomy.

Or did I wake up?

Was I in coma dreaming my life? Dreaming I'm at work, that I shaved my head, that I'm on chemo? I was tired, too tired to think.

CHAPTER EIGHT

The Note

"When you come to the end of your rope, tie a knot and hang on." — Franklin D. Roosevelt

I love summer and swimming in my pool, but I could not be in the sun for long periods of time while on chemo. Aching for some normalcy in my life, I invited my parents, my brother Steve, sister-in-law Donna, and niece Kenzie over to hang at the pool with Alex and me. I told Alex's dad, Kevin, he was welcome to join us because he was coming to visit Alex like he did most weekends anyway.

Having all of us hanging out, talking, eating, laughing was exactly what I needed. My brother was relaxing on a float with Rudy lying across him. I'm sure he felt like a wooly afghan was covering half his body, but Steve didn't seem to care. Rudy enjoyed sunbathing like the rest of us. Since it was evident Steve couldn't get up without disturbing Master Rudy, I asked him if I could bring his dessert to the pool. Steve said that would be great, so I went inside for his slice of cake. When Kevin saw me hand the plate to Steve, he yelled in his New York accent, *"Hey Steve! I couldn't get ha to do that for me even when I had a ring on ha finga!"* Everybody broke into laughter. I wanted normalcy. I got it!

Kevin and I split up when Alex was eleven months old, and we were divorced by the time she was two. He never remarried. Since my cancer diagnosis, often when he came over to see Alex, he would bring homemade food—lasagna, teriyaki chicken, pork chops—all kinds of dishes that he cooked himself. To this day, I know Kevin has a big heart, and he loves Alex. Despite our differences, I think he still loves me, too.

October

Chemo was over. I still had to take the Herceptin, and reconstructive surgery lay on the horizon, but at least I wasn't puking and my hair stopped falling out. Speaking of hair, I had only a little bit that was extremely curly; it resembled a Brillo pad. When I'm lying on the couch, the throw pillows cling to my hair like Velcro!

With my mind clear of chemo, I made a discovery. I realized that mysterious beeping I heard in my office came from the building's elevator. The noise, which signaled that the elevator had reached its weight capacity, would strangely bounce off the corridor walls, down the hall, echoing through my office.

The expander implanted during my mastectomy remained in my chest. Every month the doctor would give me a good stab with a saline-filled syringe in the breast where I had the mastectomy. The purpose was to increase the capacity of the area gradually. By slowly stretching the newly grafted skin, an implant could eventually be inserted during reconstructive surgery and the expander removed. Yep, just another day in paradise!

Do you find it a bit unnerving when doctors call what they do practice?

One of my doctors wrote an order for me to have a follow-up MRI at an Atlanta hospital. Just before I was about to get in the MRI machine, I happened to mention in a conversation with the nurse that I had an expander in my chest. She immediately stopped what she was doing and turned to me. "What kind of expander is it?" she asked.

"What kind?" I repeated. "Do you mean...brand name?"

"Yes," she replied.

I was thinking how the heck I would know what brand it is—it's not like I shopped for it at the mall! *It's a Tommy Hilfiger, but it's* so last year! *M*aybe the doctor who stuffed it into my chest cavity as I lay unconscious might be more likely to have that information?

Sure enough, after numerous calls to my team of doctors, the professionals in charge of my wellbeing determined that my expander had metal in it. One nurse then told me I could have been badly burned by the MRI. Another said the machine could have made the metal piece spin around inside me. Someone else suggested that the machine could have ripped it completely out of my chest. (Now *that* would have knocked me right out of the wet t-shirt contest I entered!)

Later, during a visit with my oncologist, I relayed what happened. He was *not* the doctor who'd sent me for the MRI. Leaning back in his chair and slowly shaking his head from side to side, he gave me a look. I'm talking about an expression on his face that said I'd come within an inch of something awful. After a moment, he said, "Lesa, I know of a situation in which a husband asked to be in the room while his wife had her MRI. No one knew that the spouse was a runner who customarily wore ankle weights. Within seconds after the machine was turned on, his ankles and legs were jerked out from under him and up into the air abruptly snapping and breaking both ankles."

After hearing that story, I must confess that from getting cancer plus having an overdose of morphine and a near miss with an MRI machine, I decided a few less brushes with death would be nice about now.

November

I had reconstructive surgery! A saline implant took the place of the expander, which had created space for my new boob! My other breast also gained a saline implant so I could have a matching pair. The procedure was to be outpatient surgery, and I was to leave the hospital after recovering for a few hours.

As my luck would have it, or should I say lack thereof, I started vomiting after the surgery, and that continued through the wee hours of the night so I wasn't allowed to leave the hospital. I was given a variety of nausea medications until they found one that worked. My retching finally subsided by morning. After that exhausting episode, they allowed me to go home.

January Next Year

Finally, I could see a flicker of light at the end of a long, snaking tunnel.

I was gaining my energy back, and food tasted good again. Months ago I had begun to sleep about five hours on my own, and that was when I had stopped taking the sleeping pills. Without the lingering effects of the sleeping pills or chemo fog, I felt clear and focused at work.

The collapsed veins in my arms were also disappearing, so I could wear short sleeves. I was exercising and beginning to feel like my old self again. Although my period disappeared after my second chemo and never came back, I honestly don't care if it ever does. (As far as I'm concerned, that's a perk of chemo!) I had a little more hair, but it was so extremely curly that it did not look like it had grown much at all. Some people say their hair has a mind of its own; well, mine has a severe personality disorder! For work I replaced the blonde wig with a black University of Georgia baseball cap.

Anyway, things were looking up until one random day I began feeling nauseated at work. I struggled to make it to the end of the work day without asking to leave early. Although I managed to stick it out until five o'clock, I was progressively getting sicker and sicker. When I got in my car to head home, I put a plastic bag in the seat beside me. I was sure I would throw up. I sat in traffic on the interstate with one hand on the steering wheel and the other gripping a Wal-Mart shopping bag. Somehow I made it home without hurling in the bag, but as soon as I ran in the door and straight to the bathroom, I threw up. Alex wasn't home so, I went in my bedroom and lay down on my bed. I went back and forth from my bed to the bathroom throwing up for five straight hours, until eleven pm. I assumed the culprit was some type of flu bug because I shouldn't have been experiencing chemo-related nausea at that point.

Feeling better but drained, I swaggered from wall to wall to the fridge in my sweats looking for water and crackers. Once in the kitchen, I saw a piece of paper on the counter with something typed on it. I picked it up, but I couldn't read the message because I didn't have my contacts in. I was so weak by this time and I had no energy at all, but I slowly walked back to my bedroom and retrieved my glasses. I began reading…

Dear Mom,

This is the hardest letter I have ever had to write. There is something I need to tell you and I am so scared and sorry for putting this on you. You have always been there for me no matter what. Through thick and thin like no one else. That's why I am coming to you to tell you that I am 5 weeks pregnant. I am so sorry. I hope you're not too disappointed in me. I never wanted this to happen or to put you through this. Today I bought pregnancy tests and they were both positive. I also went to a walk-in clinic to get an official test. I love you so much and I am so sorry! I hope that you find it in your heart to be open and forgiving. I am telling Radford tonight before church. I will be home at the regular time and we can talk about this. Just remember that this is happening to me and I am more scared than you can imagine. I need you! So, I don't know how Radford is going to handle this so please wait to talk to me until I get home. I Love you I love you I love you!!! I am so sorry!

Love,

Alex

I threw up for three more hours.

When Alex got home from church, she came to my bedroom. I was a rung out shell of human flesh. To say that I felt completely devastated and defeated in all directions of life is a gross understatement. For months I felt as though I was drowning financially, emotionally and physically, bobbing up for enough air to stay alive. This night, it felt like someone put a foot on top of my drowning head and pushed me completely under. I couldn't breathe.

CHAPTER NINE

Déjà vu

*"I know God will not give me anything
I can't handle.... I just wish that he didn't
trust me so much." – Mother Teresa*

With the news of Alex's pregnancy, I could barely function from pure despair. Alex has always been everything to me. I love her more than life itself. All I could think about were the years of raising my beautiful little girl, the five-year-old who danced the Macarena in her mother's old cocktail dress, the child that wanted to be a mermaid when she grew up. Those were the best years of my life.

One night years ago when she was about two, we sat together under her white eyelet canopy bed. I put the palms of her tiny hands together pointed up, and asked her to bow her head down and close her eyes. She did exactly as I asked. Then I told her to ask God to take care of us, and to thank Him for our food and anything else she wanted to thank Him for. She thanked Him for flowers and her cat Diamond. (Diamond is 15 years old as I write this.) From that day on, she has always prayed.

When Alex was four, she and I lived in a condominium complex where she played with kids from a variety of backgrounds. One day, as I'm watching her play through the sliding glass door, she interrupted her outdoor games to run across the courtyard to our patio. I slid open the door to see what she wanted. She had a question. "Mom, what are we?"

"What do you mean?" I asked.

"What religion are we?"

She went on to tell me she'd met some kids who said they were Jehovah's Witnesses, and she wanted to tell them what we were. I said, "We're Christian." She smiled at me with her bright eyes. "Okay," she said, immediately turning, her disheveled auburn hair flying as she ran to tell her friends. As I leaned against the doorway watching her, I wondered what other kids were told when they ask their parents that same question. I wondered what the eyes of other children looked like when their mothers or fathers replied, "Our family doesn't believe in God." I wondered how that sort of moment affected the rest of those children's lives.

We attended a local Baptist church on Sunday mornings, so most of the kids Alex knew were Protestant. Even though I didn't share the beliefs of our Jehovah's Witness neighbors, the kids and their parents were some of the nicest people I had ever met. Six well-behaved, well-mannered, sweet, home-schooled kids lived with their two parents in a two-bedroom condo.

One day I noticed one of the kids skating with only one skate on and he looked to be having fun. Alex said the boy found it and that the girls didn't have many toys. That day I asked my daughter if she'd like to gather all her Barbies that she didn't play with anymore (which was a lot) and let the five girls each pick one to keep. Alex was excited and started gathering the dolls and putting them in a pile. The neighbor girls had to obtain their mother's permission to accept a doll, so after they got her approval, all five of them came over.

I sat on the staircase above them peering through the banister to watch the girls. So happy and excited, they gathered in a circle around a pile of half-dressed Barbies. I'll never forget their faces. Each of them picked a Barbie and an outfit to take home. As they were leaving, I told them I found a pair of skates that no longer fit Alex and sent the skates with them as well. Such were the memories of Alex's life that played through my thoughts. To me, part of Alex would always be the little girl who sat under the white eyelet canopy bed wearing pink nail polish and snuggling her cat.

*"In spite of the cost of living,
it's still popular." - Kathy Norris*

Still January

I received notice in the mail that my car insurance had been cancelled on both my cars. Alex's wreck and ticket had caught up with us. Long story short, I scrambled to find another carrier. Day after day on my lunch hour, I sat in my office calling insurance companies for quotes or researching and disputing a medical bill. Neulasta, one of the shots I had to take with chemo, carried a per unit price tag of nearly six grand. What the heck does the syringe have in it—diamonds? Eventually, I found new car insurance, but it was off-the-charts expensive. I realized that the underwriters viewed Alex as a risk, but you could insure a small country for what it was costing me to cover her! I had no choice. It was the only company that would take us, therefore adding to my financial pressure. I felt caught in a vice with the air literally being squeezed out of me.

Still reeling from the shock of Alex's pregnancy and juggling one issue after another on the phone at work during lunch, I could at least keep in mind that I was nearing the end of my Herceptin treatment. I hoped never to see the inside of a chemo room again. Those exact thoughts were interrupted by my vibrating cell phone.

"Hello?"

"Is this Lesa?" the woman asked.

"Yes," I said.

"Lesa, this is Dr. Auda's office. Dr. Auda needs to speak with you. Can you hold?"

Dear God, you've seriously got to be kidding me. As a matter of fact, no, no I don't want to hold for Dr Auda!

"Yes I'll hold," I replied.

"Hello, is this Lesa?" Doctor Auda asked.

"Yes, hi Doctor Auda."

He was calling to tell me that my recent routine mammogram showed there may be cancer in my other breast. What do you know? A mammogram was finally doing its job.

And by the way, could somebody wake me from this "Nightmare on Déjà Vu Street"!

Dr. Auda's office scheduled me for a biopsy. The procedure was uncomfortable, painful, but not unbearable. After, I had dressed, paid my insurance co-payment, and started to leave, a nurse asked me to wait a minute. I complied and she called me back to a room. The technician told me that the tiny metal marker that had been injected into my breast during the biopsy did not show up in the x-ray.

So I asked, "Well, where is it?"

The technician didn't know.

"What do you mean you don't know? Is it floating around in my rib cage somewhere?"

The staff assured me that it wasn't displaced in my body. Most likely, the ejecting instrument used during the biopsy malfunctioned so that the metal marker never entered my body.

Well, of course, the instrument malfunctioned! Would somebody please just shoot me now? Never mind….. The gun would probably jam.

Back down on the table, I was poked and prodded a second time. I don't think I'm out of line to say that the words *black* and *cloud* came to mind. Even so, if this shit didn't hurt so badly, I almost would have laughed at the irony.

I bled through the gauze, into my bra during the entire hour and a half drive home. My bra was saturated with blood and my breast was badly bruised black, blue, purple and yellow for a month.

I was later notified that the biopsy found no trace of cancer. So much for thinking I'd finally had a mammogram that did its job. Remind me again where I put my Polaroid camera.

CHAPTER TEN

Blue Eyes

"Breathe. Let go. And remind yourself that this very moment is the only one you know you have for sure." — Oprah Winfrey

Hostility, tears, arguments and controversy surrounded Alex's pregnancy. Some of her friends had undergone abortions; a few of them told her that's what she needed to do, others told her she would regret it forever if she did. Some thought she should marry the father and keep the baby since they were in love and had been together for more than two years. Every person has an abortion opinion, and a pregnant teenager can find plenty of people to tell her what she should or should not do.

College and bright future that had been awaiting her seemed to be vanishing. If she kept the baby, was she throwing her life away? She'd already been accepted to college and was set to start in the fall. Her dad and I had been saving for her college since she was two, and she'd looked forward to going for as long as any of us could remember. However, from the time it took her to write her apology note and leave it on the kitchen counter, a moral dilemma loomed.

I was in pain from despair from the time I found out she was pregnant. I'm not speaking metaphorically; I actually felt physical pain from the heartache of learning that she was pregnant. All the while, I was still on cancer treatments and covered up in bills.

After much soul searching…

Alex graduated with her High School Senior class in the spring. She went on to excel in college. As I finish this manuscript, she is a junior studying journalism at the University of Georgia with a bright wonderful future in front of her. Alex has demonstrated a writing talent since childhood. But that's not all.

Alex asked me very early in her pregnancy if I thought a soul was already inside of her at that point. She said she was being bombarded with all kinds of opinions. I told her yes, but I assured her that the only opinion that mattered was the Creator of souls. So she took her research to the Bible and here is what she found: *"Before I formed you in the womb, I knew you…."* (Jeremiah 1:5)

Thus…

Baby boy Tristen David Radford arrived on earth in September. His eight pounds, ten ounces of perfection came with bright blue eyes and a dimpled chin. Alex loves him beyond words, as does our entire family. She matured quickly from here, and, above all, neither Alex nor I have ever regretted her decision to have her baby boy, keep him and raise him. She has been as good a mother to Tristen from the time he was born as I was to her at twenty-seven.

Alex and Tristen live with me, so I see firsthand that

she manages her responsibilities as a fulltime student and parents like an old pro.

The girl can simultaneously change a diaper, wipe a runny nose, text two friends, and rehearse a speech for class out loud while dispensing animal crackers as she listens to the tunes of Rascal Flatts while watching the MTV music awards. All this while wearing an applesauce covered Ed Hardy T-shirt.

But there were times when her naiveté had a bazaar twist of humor. When she was packing for the hospital, she stuffed her clothes in her school backpack instead of in a suitcase. I insisted that she use one of the many proper pieces of luggage that we owned. Later, when I went to see what she had packed, I found that she considered her cheerleading duffel bag to be appropriate baggage. This one sported her name cheerfully embroidered alongside a large megaphone.

The hospital essentials that she packed included five movies to watch. Fortunately, she asked me which of her most comfortable t-shirts she should take. Like many teens, Alex reminded me that she didn't own an actual nightgown. Thus, among the choices she presented were a Rolling Stones number with that famous tongue on the front (nice visual on a nine-months-pregnant teenager, huh?), her High School "Senior Class of 2007" shirt (might as well wear a billboard and announce you're a teen mother), and her "Jesus Is My Homeboy" t-shirt with Jesus' face front and center. (I can't even comment by now, I'm just rubbing my temples!)

Geez…this is going to be a long eighteen years ahead of us!

That being said, life has moved on. It's been five years since I had breast cancer. I'm due another Polaroid—I mean *mammogram*—in six months. However, I'm thinking of using a more accurate, scientific method to detect breast cancer this time. I'm going to lie down and let a large Collie walk across my chest!

Alex and Tristen's father are still happily together and have a wedding planned for this year.

Looking back, I see that when I couldn't change my circumstances, I *could* change my perspective. And neither we nor our children are perfect, but God is.

As for you out there who are overwhelmed with circumstances in your own life, laugh at yourself when you can, and most of all, know that you're not alone.

It's just one of those *daze!*

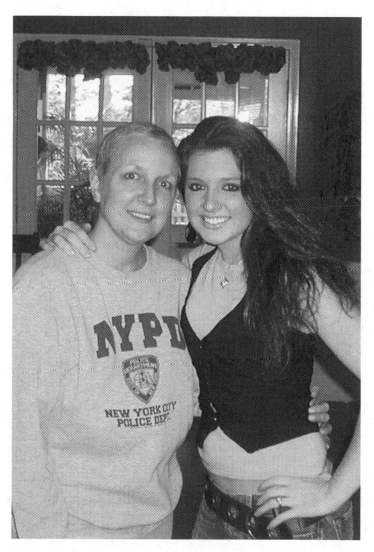

Lesa & Alex

About the Author

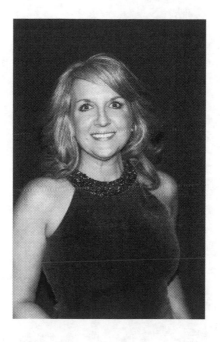

Born and raised in Gainesville, Georgia, Lesa Osborn attended the University of Georgia and later worked as a Flight Attendant. At the time of her breast cancer diagnosis, she was employed by a national real estate publishing company. Today, Lesa owns a photography business and resides in Suwanee, Georgia. Sharing her story from a humorous perspective, she accepts speaking engagements.

www.365DazeBook.com